TOAST
&
TRAINERS

EATING WELL AS A STUDENT

Kate Birch-Scanlan
BSc(hons) NTDip

Disclaimer
The information in this book is intended to provide useful information on the subjects discussed. This book is not meant to be used nor should it be used to diagnose or treat any medical condition. Consult your own physician for any diagnosis or medical treatment of a problem.

The publisher and author are not responsible for any specific health or allergy needs that may require supervision and are not liable for any damages or negative consequences that may occur to any person reading or following the information in this book.

References provided are for informal purposes only.

This is for you our Joe.

We know cooking will not be at the top of your list of things to do whilst you are away studying unless you unleash a new passion.
So, we wrote you this book to help you out. It contains easy meals with minimal mess and washing up, cheap recipes, and meal plans to help you feel healthy whilst you are busy embarking on the next stage in your life.

Love Mum and E xx

CONTENTS

INTRODUCTION

Moving away from home when you are a teenager to go to university, college or set up on your own is an exciting time. Making new friends and having the freedom to do whatever you want, whenever you want.

You are likely to be taking on more responsibility for your own wellbeing than you have ever done before. It can be quite daunting to take responsibility for your own food shopping, washing, cleaning, and planning.

This book is to help you with the food shopping and meal planning part, as it is likely that you won't want to spend time cooking and washing up, you'll be far too busy for that!!

It shows you how to cheaply and effortlessly get the nutrients that your brain and gut require to stay as well as possible.

If you make the effort to include more of certain foods in your diet you will feel better both physically and mentally. You will have more energy, better concentration, sleep better, have better gut health and be more resilient.

Important Nutrients

Omega 3 – Omega 3 fatty acids are vital for the brain and nervous system. They are essential for maintaining the insulating sleeve which surrounds nerves called the myelin sheath, allowing signals to flow down the nerves at the right speed. Omega 3 fatty acids reduce inflammation. Inflammation is connected to many health issues including mental ill health.
It is found in oily fish such as salmon, mackerel, and sardines. Vegans may require a supplement from an algae source.

Zinc – Zinc helps our bodies deal with stress. Clinical studies have shown that zinc levels appear to be lower in people who are anxious or depressed.
Food sources include beef, pork, beans, cashew nuts, chickpeas, pumpkin seeds, walnuts, prawn, green leafy vegetables, lentils, tofu, and sesame seeds.

Magnesium – Magnesium works with calcium to relax muscles. It is important for the management of stress, anxiety, and depression. It helps relax muscle tension and helps you to unwind. It also can aid sleep and reduces pain in aching joints and muscles.
Good food sources include green leafy vegetables, avocados, bananas, nuts, seeds, wholegrains and dark chocolate.

Calcium – As mentioned above it works with magnesium to relax you. It is important for regulating mood and for good bone health.
Food sources include, dairy products, fortified plant milks, almonds, green leafy vegetables, broccoli, and parsley.

B vitamins – This is a group of vitamins that are essential to wellbeing. They are water soluble so they cannot be stored by the body therefore, you need to eat them every day. They are the key components of energy production and support the nervous system. Low levels of certain B vitamins have been linked to mental health conditions such as depression and anxiety.

To keep your B vitamin levels topped up include whole grains such as brown rice, oats, quinoa, barley and whole wheat foods, green vegetables, oily fish, and meat.

Vitamin D – There is a connection between low levels of vitamin D and low mood. Having low levels of vitamin D is not good for your gut health and can lead to inflammation in the body which has been linked to depression and other mental health conditions. Vitamin D is also essential for your immune system.
To increase your vitamin D intake, get out in the sunshine if you can, eat mushrooms, eggs and take a supplement from October through to March of 10 micrograms.

Vitamin C – Vitamin C helps protect cells and keep them healthy. It also helps to keep skin healthy, maintain bones and cartilage and help with wound healing.
It is found in a variety of fruits and vegetables. Good sources include citrus fruits, peppers, strawberries, blackcurrants, broccoli and potatoes.

Fibre – Scientific understanding of the connection between our brain and our gut has increased over recent years. Fibre has been shown to be a very beneficial component when it comes to improving gut health and reducing stress.
Research has shown that people eating a diet containing plenty of fibrous foods are likely to experience less stress and anxiety.
Adding some fibrous foods to each meal such as fruits, vegetables, pulses, nuts, seeds, whole grains and oats is the easiest way to increase your fibre intake.

Water – Our brains are made up of about 75% water and are dependent on proper hydration to function properly.
If we don't drink enough water, we can have difficulty concentrating, get headaches, brain fog and changes in mood. Your short-term and long-term memory can also be impacted.
Studies have shown that loss of water as little as 1.5% can alter a person's energy levels and mood. It is recommended that we drink at least 2 litres of water a day. A red flag for dehydration is darker urine.

Look After Your Gut Health and Your Gut Will Look After You

To look after your physical health you probably already know that you need to have healthy eating habits, but are you aware of the role that nutrition plays in brain health and the maintenance of our mental well-being?

The impact that food has on our brain is gradual and builds up over time. Therefore, eating well for brain health requires us to build up regular long-term habits.

The energy that our brain uses is about 25% of our daily energy requirement. It uses vitamins and minerals in all its cellular activity. So, if you start to run low on nutrients your brain will begin to struggle and as your brain is in charge or your thoughts and feelings it is a good idea to feed it properly.

If you want to take care of your brain the best thing that you can do is take care of your gut.

The gut and brain communicate via the vagus nerve, the communication is bidirectional, so the brain can influence the gut and the gut can shape the brain.

Bacteria, viruses and fungi that live in the gut known as the gut microbiome synthesise compounds that travel to the brain in the bloodstream and influence brain health and activity.

Problems with digestion may deplete the brain of nutrients that it requires to function properly.

If the gut wall becomes damaged through poor nutrition systematic inflammation can occur in the body which may harm the brain and have and effect on our mental health.

To take care of your gut:

- Include more fibre such as wholemeal bread, whole wheat pasta, beans, lentils, roasted vegetables and potatoes with the skins on.
- Include plenty of leafy greens and salads.
- Add oily fish to meals such as mackerel, sardines and salmon.
- Drink plenty of water.
- Get enough vitamin D from eggs, mushrooms, sunshine and a supplement in the autumn and winter months.
- Consume a diverse range of foods in the form of fruits, vegetables, nuts, seeds, healthy fats and wholegrains. A variety of these types of foods is key because these foods feed the 'beneficial' bacteria in our gut which help keep our brains and body healthy.
- Include live yogurt (unsweetened) and fermented foods such as kimchi, sauerkraut and kombucha which contain probiotic bacteria which are beneficial to the gut.

Foods to Limit to Maintain a Healthy Gut Include:

- Alcohol
- Caffeine
- Sugar
- Artificial sweeteners
- Emulsifiers - Added to pre-packaged foods to prevent fats and lipids from separating.
- Too many takeaways

"It's about eating well enough; you don't need to be perfect".

Where Do I Begin?

Moving away from home can be an emotional time. Try your best to eat well and sleep well to stay healthy. Keep food familiar, simple to prepare, accessible and filling. It is about eating 'well enough' but not trying to be too perfect.

Quick and Familiar Main Meal Ideas

Soup with Bread and Butter – Go for soups with vegetables in plus beans, rice or lentils.

Tinned Mackerel, Mixed Frozen or Tinned Vegetables, Brown Rice and Nandos Peri Peri Sauce.

Scrambled Egg on Toast with Watercress.

Tuna and Pesto Toastie with Cherry Tomatoes.

Cooked Chicken, Mixed Nuts, Lettuce, Tomato and Cucumber.

Stir Fry, Cashew Nuts and Noodles.

Fish Finger and Salad Sandwiches (using wholemeal bread).

Pasta, Vegan Pesto and Vegan Cheese.

Jacket Potato with Tuna and Sweetcorn or Baked Beans and Cheese.

Beans on Wholemeal Toast with Grated Cheese.

Tip: Add salad foods to meals to add extra nutrients, they take very little time to prepare and wash up and they can make you feel more alert and clearer headed.

Tastes Homemade
(but quicker and cheaper)

Quick and Easy Chilli and Brown Rice
Ingredients:
1 tin of black beans
1 tin of kidney beans
1 tin of chopped tomatoes
Chilli flakes to taste – approximately 1 teaspoon
1 sachet of brown rice
Grated cheese

Put all the ingredients in a saucepan and leave to cook for 20 minutes.
Serve with Brown rice, cheese.

Egg Fried Rice
Ingredients:
1 sachet of brown rice
Frozen mixed vegetables
2 eggs
Tamari/soy sauce

Put a tablespoon of olive oil in a frying pan and heat.
Add 2 cups of mixed frozen vegetables to the frying pan and cook until piping hot.
Heat the rice in the microwave.
Break the eggs into a cup and whisk.
Add the egg to the vegetables in the frying pan and stir with a wooden spoon until the egg is mixed through the vegetables and turns into a scrambled egg consistency.
Add the cooked rice and stir.
Add a sprinkling of tamari sauce.

Tip: Tinned, frozen and fresh fruit and vegetables are all nutritious, so don't feel like you have to buy fresh if it's easier for you to buy frozen or tinned options.

Shopping List

Main Meals:
Wholemeal Bread
Margarine
Brown Rice
Brown Rice Pasta (or whole wheat pasta)
Eggs
Tuna
Tinned Mackerel
Frozen Fish Fingers
Cashew Nuts
Mixed Nuts
Noodles
Baked Beans
Black Beans
Kidney Beans
Tinned Chopped Tomatoes
Tinned Soup (with vegetables and beans, lentils or rice)
Chilli Flakes
Vegan Cheese (non-vegan if you eat dairy)
Jacket Potatoes
Vegan Pesto (non-vegan if you eat dairy)
Cooked Chicken (or raw to cook yourself)
Lettuce
Tomatoes
Cucumber
Watercress
Breakfast and Lunches:
Breakfast Cereal (lower sugar ones like Weetabix, Shredded Wheat, and Bran flakes)
Plant based (eg soya) Live Yogurts
Fruit – bananas, apples, pears, plums, oranges and kiwis all store well.
Peanut Butter
Marmite
Dark Chocolate
Plant Based Milk (or milk if you eat dairy)
Tea/coffee

2 MEAL PLANS AND SHOPPING LISTS

Once you have found your feet, you could adapt them, or create your own.

Meal Plan 1

	Breakfast	Lunch	Dinner
Monday	**Weetabix and soya milk.**	**Marmite Sandwich on Wholemeal Bread.** Apple and pear. Nuts.	**Mackerel and Rice -** Tinned or smoked mackerel, sachet brown rice, tin of peas, tin of sweetcorn, Nandos sauce. Heat the rice and tinned vegetables in the microwave and mix together. Add the mackerel on top and a drizzle of Nandos sauce.
Tuesday	**Yogurt and a piece of fruit.**	**Peanut Butter Wrap.** Apple. Dark chocolate. (Save some wraps for dinner tomorrow night!)	**Tuna, Pesto, and Cheese Toastie** on wholemeal bread with chopped tomato and cucumber. Mix the tuna and some pesto together in a bowl. Place on the bread with a sprinkling of cheese. Cook in the toastie machine. Serve with tomatoes and cucumber or watercress.
Wednesday	**Shredded Wheat** with soya milk	**Buy lunch out** (or make a sandwich, plus fruit)	**Rice, Bean, Lettuce, Tomato and Cheese Wrap** Heat the rice and beans in the microwave and mix together. Heat the wrap for a few seconds. Add to a wrap some of the beans, rice, some

	Breakfast	Lunch	Dinner
			shredded lettuce, chopped tomato, jalapenos and cheese then fold into a wrap.
Thursday	**Yogurt and Fruit.**	**Marmite Sandwich,** fruit, vegetable sticks, dark chocolate.	**Tinned chicken curry and brown rice with salad.**
Friday	**Weetabix** and soya milk.	**Peanut Butter Sandwich,** fruit, dark chocolate etc.	**Tinned Chilli and Brown Rice.**
Saturday	**Cereal/ Toast/Yogurt.**	**Toastie** Tuna, pesto, cheese.	**Jacket Potato, Beans, and Cheese.**
Sunday	**Cereal/ Toast/Yogurt.**	**Scrambled Egg on Wholemeal Toast.**	**Chicken, Tofu, or Cashew Nut Stir fry with Noodles.** Use pre-prepared stir fry vegetables. Fry chicken, tofu, or cashew nuts in a little olive oil in a frying pan then remove from the frying pan. Cook the stir fry in a little olive oil in the frying pan. Whilst the stir fry is cooking cook the noodles as instructed on the packet. Mix the vegetables, meat/nuts and noodles together and sprinkle a

			little tamari or soy sauce on top. *For more flavour add some chopped chilli.* OR M&S Balanced ready meal.

I have used marmite and peanut butter for the sandwiches as they are store cupboard essentials in our house and do not go off quickly, therefore ideal for student life and to keep cost down. Feel free to use alternative fillings.

Tip: Snack on fruit and vegetable sticks like celery, cucumber and carrots to increase your fruit and vegetable intake and reduce sugar and fat consumption from processed and convenience foods.

Over time aim to increase the variety of vegetables that you add to your meals if you can. Check out the offers for the week in the supermarket and be creative.

Turn to page 35 for salad ideas.

Shopping List for Meal Plan 1

Work through the list and write down which foods you need to buy this week. Remember there are some foods that will last potentially for several weeks such as margarine and peanut butter, so some weeks your shop will cost more than others.

4 sachets of brown rice
2 tins of tuna
Loaf of wholemeal bread
Tomatoes
Cucumber
Margarine
Marmite
Peanut butter
Tinned peas
Tinned sweetcorn
Vegan pesto
Vegan cheese
Smoked mackerel
Eggs
Jacket potatoes
Baked beans
Jalapeno peppers
Tinned curry
Tinned chilli
Nandos sauce
Stir fry vegetables
Noodles
Cashew nuts
Yogurts
Tamari
Fruits of your choice
Dark chocolate
Weetabix

Shredded wheat
Soya milk (Unsweetened and fortified)
Wraps
Margarine
Coffee
Ginger tea
Smoothies

Meal Plan 2

	Breakfast	Lunch	Dinner
Monday	**Cereal –** Weetabix, Shredded Wheat or Bran flakes, anything with a lower sugar content.	**Nut Butter Wrap**. Fruit. Dark chocolate.	**Pitta, Beans, Rice and Houmous.** Heat the rice and beans thoroughly. Add to a toasted pitta. Add salad and houmous. Save left over pittas for Tuesday's lunch.
Tuesday	**Yogurt and Fruit.**	**Ham or Cheese Salad Pitta** (use up pittas from previously night). Fruit. Nuts.	**Pasta, Pesto, Tuna, Sweetcorn, and Cheese.** Cook the pasta and run under cold water. In a pan heat olive oil and a spoonful of pesto, then add tuna and sweetcorn. Heat thoroughly. Heat the pasta in the microwave and mix with the pesto. Sprinkle on a little cheese.
Wednesday	**Marmite on Wholemeal Toast.**	**Buy Lunch Out.**	**Beans on Wholemeal Toast.** Followed by some fruit.
Thursday	**Cereal.**	**Nut Butter Sandwich.** Fruit or chopped vegetable sticks. Dark Chocolate	**Mackerel, Brown rice, and Vegetables.** Heat the rice, then heat a tin of mixed vegetables and mix in the rice. Add the mackerel on top and some Nandos

			sauce.
Friday	**Yogurt and Fruit.**	**Marmite Sandwich.** Dark chocolate. Banana.	**Tinned Chilli and Brown rice.**
Saturday	**Nut Butter on Toast.**	**Tuna Pesto Toastie**	**Scrambled Eggs, with Spinach, Tomatoes, and Wholemeal Pittas.** Wisk 2 eggs in a cup. Heat a teaspoon of olive oil in a saucepan. When hot pour the egg into the pan. Add a handful of spinach, mix in and cook through. Serve with some chopped tomatoes in a couple of toasted wholemeal pittas.
Sunday	**Yogurt and fruit**	**Peanut Butter Wrap,** (save some wraps for Mondays lunchbox).	**Jacket Potato, Tuna, and Cucumber.** Cook the potato in the microwave or oven. Mix the tuna with a little mayonnaise and finely chopped cucumber. Add the tuna/cucumber to the potato. Serve with extra salad for more nutrients.

Tip: Snack on foods like nuts, vegetable sticks and houmous, pittas and houmous, rice cakes and houmous, oatcakes, hard boiled eggs and fruit such as bananas, apple, pears and oranges.

Shopping List for Meal Plan 2

Check through the following list and make a list of what you need to get in your weekly food shop for this meal plan.

Breakfast cereal -Weetabix, Shredded Wheat, Bran flakes etc……….
Soya milk (unsweetened and fortified)
Peanut Butter
Marmite
Wholemeal Bread
Margarine
2 packs of pitta bread (freeze one if date is short)
Houmous
Salad leaves
Tomatoes
Cucumber
Tinned or frozen mixed vegetables
Tinned sweetcorn
Brown rice pasta (or whole wheat pasta)
Brown rice (3 sachets of pre prepared rice or 1 bag of uncooked rice)
Vegan cheese
Vegan pesto
Baked beans
Tinned chilli
Tinned mackerel
2 tins of tuna
Eggs
Frozen or fresh spinach
Jacket Potato
Wraps
Live yogurts
Your choice of fruits
Nandos sauce
Olive oil
Dark chocolate
Nuts for snacks
Ginger teabags

Shopping Tips

Fruit

When you buy fruit firstly look for what is on offer, usually at the end of the fruit aisle.

Also, go for fruits that last longer such as apples, pears, oranges, kiwis, and fruits that say ripen at home.

Frozen fruits are useful to add to yogurt, porridge, ice cream and smoothies, or on their own.

Do not dismiss tinned fruit, just make sure it is in natural juice and not syrup. Tinned fruit is a really good way to increase your fruit intake without having to keep going to the shops!

Include a couple of pieces of fruit every day.

Vegetables

As with fruit, look out for what is on offer.

Fresh, frozen, and tinned are all great.

Add tinned or frozen vegetables such as peas, sweetcorn, and carrots to rice.

If you have no time to cook, buy cucumber, tomatoes and little gem lettuces which require minimal preparation.

Try and have some vegetables everyday with your evening meal.

Rice

Go for brown basmati rice or wholegrain rice.

If you are stuck for time microwavable sachets of precooked rice are useful, just remember larger bags of uncooked rice are more cost effective.

To jazz things up a bit buy sachets of rice with quinoa, lentils or chickpeas.

Soups

Buy soups which contain several vegetables. Also, to make them more filling and provide extra fibre look out for soups which contain lentils or rice.

Fish

Tinned, frozen and fresh fish are all good for you.
Tinned fish stores for longer and keeps the cost down.
Try to include some oily fish in your diet each week for brain health, such as mackerel, sardines, or salmon.
Tinned or fresh smoked mackerel is lovely added to rice. Tinned sardines taste great on wholemeal toast.
Tuna is an easy fish to include. It is great in sandwiches, jacket potatoes/sweet potatoes, pasta, toasties, or salads.

Breakfast Cereals

Avoid sugary cereals. Go for cereals such as Weetabix, Shredded Wheat, All bran, Bran flakes or porridge which are not full of sugar and contain plenty of fibre.

Plant Milks

As you may not be getting enough nutrients go for plant milks which are fortified with calcium, vitamin B12 and vitamin D. Choose the unsweetened version.

Always try and buy shops own brand as these are often much cheaper than the well-known brands.

RECIPES

BREAKFASTS
&
SMOOTHIES

Speedy Breakfasts

It is important to eat a nutritious breakfast, even if you take it out of the door with you.
It will help you to maintain your mood, concentration, and energy levels by keeping your blood sugars levels more stable.

- Oat cakes with nut butter.
- Peanut butter and banana on toast.
- Marmite sandwich, piece of fruit and a handful of nuts.
- Chopped fruit and plain yogurt (add oats for extra fibre).
- Low sugar cereal such as Weetabix, Bran flakes or Shredded wheat. Add some chopped fruit to get extra vitamins and fibre.
- Peanut butter wrap, and a piece of fruit.

Porridge *(Serves 1)*

Ingredients
½ cup of porridge oats
1 cup of any plant milk
½ cup frozen blueberries – defrosted (save the blueberry juice!)
Mixed nuts finely chopped

Step 1
Add the porridge oats and milk to a saucepan and simmer for 5 minutes.

Step 2
Put the porridge in a bowl, top with the blueberries including the juice that comes from them and sprinkle chopped nuts on the top.

Poached Egg and Avocado on Toast *(Serves 1)*

Ingredients
2 eggs
1 avocado
2 slices of seeded bread

Step 1
Fill a small saucepan with water and bring to the boil.

Step 2
Peel and destone the avocado and cut into slices.

Step 3
Crack the egg into a cup and tip into the boiling water, then do the same with the second egg. Bring to the boil, then simmer for two minutes. Whilst the eggs are poaching toast the bread, once toasted butter the bread.

Step 4
Put the slices of avocado on the toast then top with the poach eggs.

Pineapple and Mango Smoothie *(Serves 1)*

Ingredients
1 Cup of frozen pineapple
1 cup frozen mango
1 cup Coconut milk
Mint leaves

Step 1
Allow the pineapple and mango to defrost so that it is only partially frozen.

Step 2
Add the fruit to the blender and pour over the coconut milk and add a couple of mint leaves.

Step 3
Blend until smooth. If it is too thick add some more coconut milk.

No Mess Juice *(Serves 1)*

Ingredients
Purchase one bottle of each of the following three juices for this recipe:
Beetroot juice
Carrot juice
Apple juice

1 lemon (optional)
2cm cube ginger (optional)

Step 1
Pour equal quantities of the beetroot juice, carrot juice and apple juice into a glass, saving the rest of the juice in the bottles for the following couple of days.

Step 2 (Optional)
Squeeze in the juice of one lemon. Using a garlic press squeeze the juice out of the ginger into the juice.

Blueberry, Spinach & Almond Milk Smoothie

(Serves 1)

Ingredients
1 cup frozen blueberries
1 cup almond milk
Handful of washed spinach leaves

Step 1
Allow the blueberries to defrost a little.

Step 2
Add the blueberries, almond milk and spinach to a blender and blend until smooth. If too thick add some more almond milk.

Avocado, Cucumber, Lemon and Mint Smoothie *(Serves 1)*

Ingredients
1/3 of a cucumber – chopped
1 avocado
Juice of 1 lemon
3-4 mint leaves
1 cup water

Step 1
Chop the cucumber and peel and destone the avocado.

Step 2
Put the avocado, cucumber, lemon juice, mint leaves and water in a blender and blend until smooth. If too thick add some more water.

MAIN MEALS

Salads

Salads are a good way of getting many important nutrients into your body in one meal, plus they require little or no cooking.

When making salads think of the components that you want to use. I like to get ideas by picking from the following columns, but it really is up to you what you choose.

GREEN LEAVES	SALAD VEGETABLES/HERBS	MEAT/FISH/NUTS /SEEDS/GRAINS /PULSES	FERMENTED FOODS AND PICKLES	DRESSING
Lettuce Spinach Watercress Raw Cabbage	Cucumber Tomatoes Celery Radish Broccoli Spring Onion Peppers Carrots Parsley Coriander Olives Avocado Chilli Ginger Garlic	Chicken Prawns Mackerel/Tuna Salmon Cashew Nuts Walnuts Peanuts Pumpkin Seeds Sesame Seeds Brown Rice Quinoa Lentils Chickpeas Beans	Kimchi Sauerkraut Pickled vegetables	*Sort of French Dressing!* 2 tbsp olive oil 1 tbsp white wine vinegar 1 tsp Dijon mustard. Mixed together *Lemon dressing* 2 tbsp Olive oil 1 tbsp Lemon juice Salt and pepper. Mixed together

Chickpea Stew *(Serves 2)*

Ingredients
1 large onion diced
1 tbsp olive oil
1 pepper thinly sliced
2 cloves garlic - minced
1 tin chickpeas
1 tin chopped tomatoes
1 tbsp tomato puree
2 balls of frozen spinach
1-2 tsp smoked paprika
1 tsp chilli powder
Salt and pepper

Step 1
Add the diced onion and sliced peppers to a large pan and cook in the olive oil until soft.
Step 2
Add the minced garlic and cook for a further 3 minutes.
Step 3
Wash the chickpeas and place in the pan, then add the smoked paprika and chilli powder.
Step 4
Once heated through add the tomatoes and the tomato puree.
Step 5
Once heated through, add the spinach.
Step 6
Simmer for 15 minutes.
Step 7
Add salt and pepper to taste.

Tuna, Pesto and Cheese Toastie *(Serves 1)*

Ingredients
2 slices wholemeal bread
2 tbsp vegan pesto
1 tin tuna
Grated vegan cheese (optional)

Step 1
Place the tuna in a bowl and stir in the pesto.

Step 2
Butter the outside of both slices of bread.

Step 3
On the inside of one slice of bread put the tuna and pesto.

Step 4
Sprinkle the cheese on the top of the tuna.

Step 5
Place the other slice of bread on the top, butter side up and place in the toastie machine until cooked.

Cheese Omelette, Watercress & Cucumber *(Serves 1)*

Ingredients
2-3 eggs
Grated vegan cheese
Watercress
Cucumber
Olive oil

Step 1
Crack the eggs into a cup and whisk together with a fork.

Step 2
Put 2 tsp of olive oil in a frying pan. When hot pour in the egg and move the pan around so the egg covers the bottom of the pan.

Step 3
Cook until firm then add the grated cheese and cook through so the cheese melts.

Step 4
Place the omelette on a plate along with a handful of watercress and some slices of cucumber.

To bulk it out and add more nutrients you could add cooked peppers, mushrooms, onions, spinach, or any other vegetables you like to the omelette.

Tuna Pesto Pasta *(Serves 1)*

Ingredients

¼ of a bag (approximately 125g) brown rice pasta
Tin of tuna - drained
2 tbsp vegan pesto
Vegan cheese grated
Tin of sweetcorn - drained
1 tbsp olive oil

Step 1
Cook the brown rice pasta according to the instructions on the packet, drain and run under cold water.

Step 2
Heat the olive oil in a pan and add the tuna.

Step 3
Once the tuna has heated through, add the pesto and sweetcorn and cook through. Take the pan off the heat.

Step 4
Heat the pasta in the microwave and add it to the pan, mixing together the pasta and tuna pesto. Then serve.

Stuffed Peppers *(Serves 2)*

Ingredients
2 peppers (yellow, orange, or red)
½ cup of uncooked brown rice
1 tin of black beans
4 cloves garlic
1 tsp chilli flakes
3 tsp coriander
1 tsp cumin
Olive oil

Mint yogurt:
Fresh mint
Plain soya yogurt

Step 1
Cook the brown rice as directed on the packet.

Step 2
Whilst the rice is cooking heat the oven to 200°C

Step 3
Cut the peppers in half longways and remove the seeds. Sprinkle a little olive oil on a baking tray, place on the pepper halves and cook in the oven for 15 minutes.

Step 4
Whilst the peppers are cooking, drain and wash the black beans and put in a saucepan with a drizzle of olive oil. Add the garlic, chilli flakes, coriander and cumin, mix and heat until the beans begin to break down.

Step 5
Add the rice to the bean mixture and stir together. Then scoop the mixture into the partially cooked pepper halves.

Step 6
Put the peppers back in the oven and cook for a further 10 minutes.

Step 7
Add some grated cheese (vegan) and cook for a further 5 minutes.
Whilst the peppers are in the oven finely chop some fresh mint and mix
it with 4 tablespoons of plain soya yogurt to make a mint yogurt
dressing.

Serve with a green salad and some mint yogurt.

Nachos *(Serves 2)*

Ingredients
1 bag of lightly salted tortilla chips
1 tin refried of beans
2-3 tomatoes - diced
1 onion diced
Jar of jalapeno peppers
Vegan cheese

Step 1
Heat oven to 200°C
Spread the tortilla chips evenly on a baking tray.

Step 2
Spread the refried beans over the tortilla chips, do not worry about being perfect.

Step 3
Sprinkle the diced onion, tomato, and some jalapeno peppers on top.

Step 4
Finally, sprinkle a good layer of grated cheese over the top and heat in the oven for 7-8 minutes.

Serve with salsa and some chopped avocado for extra flavour.

Avocado on Toasted Topped with Mixed Seeds *(Serves 1)*

Ingredients
2 slices of wholemeal bread
1 ripe avocado
2 tsp mixed seeds

Step 1
Toast the bread

Step 2
Whilst bread is toasting slice the avocado.

Step 3
Evenly place the avocado on the toast and sprinkle the mixed seeds over the top.

Fajitas *(serves 2)*

Ingredients
2 onions sliced
2 peppers sliced
2 cloves garlic - finely diced
1 chilli finely cut
2 chicken breasts diced
Olive oil
Wraps

Guacamole:
1 avocado
½ red onion
1 tomato
1 chilli
½ lemon

Plus:
Tomato salsa
Jalapeno peppers
Lettuce finely sliced
Grated cheese

Step 1
Fry the onion and pepper in a little olive oil until soft. Add the garlic and chilli and cook through.

Step 2
In a separate frying pan cook the chicken in a little oil.

Step 3
Add the chicken to the peppers and onions.

Step 4
To make the guacamole:
Finely dice the onion and tomato and thinly chop the chilli. Mash the avocado in a bowl and mix with the onion, tomato, and chilli. Add a small squirt of lemon juice.

Step 5
To make the fajita:
Heat a wrap in the microwave for 20 seconds.
Place a spoonful of the chicken, pepper, and onion mixture in the centre of a wrap.

Add some guacamole, tomato salsa, cheese, and jalapeno peppers.
Fold in the ends of the wrap, roll and enjoy.

Fancy Eggy Bread *(Serves 1)*

Ingredients
2 slices wholemeal bread
2 eggs
Olive oil
Green salad leaves or watercress
Tomatoes

Step 1
Cut the bread up into quarters.

Step 2
Crack the eggs into a bowl and whisk up using a fork.

Step 3
Place half of the bread quarters in the egg, leave for a few minutes then turn them over and leave for another few minutes.

Step 4
Heat approximately 1 tbsp of olive oil in a frying pan. Then place the egg-soaked bread quarters in the frying pan and fry until golden brown. Once brown turn them over and cook the other side. Once cooked remove from the pan and place under foil to remain warm.

Step 5
Soak the left-over bread quarters in the whisked egg and repeat step 4.

Step 6
Finally serve the eggy bread with a side of salad leaves or watercress and some sliced tomato.

Mackerel, Egg and Brown Rice *(Serves 1-2)*

Ingredients

1 sachet of brown rice
Mackerel either tinned or pre-cooked refrigerated
2 hard-boiled eggs
1 small tin of sweetcorn
1 tin of peas or frozen peas
Nandos sauce
Extra salad or vegetables such as tomatoes, cucumber, green salad leaves or broccoli.

Step 1
Heat the rice in the microwave.

Step 2
Whilst the rice is cooking heat the peas and sweetcorn in a saucepan and drain.

Step 3
Mix the rice, peas, and sweetcorn together in a bowl.

Step 4
Slice up the eggs, flake the mackerel and place on top of the rice.

Step 5
Drizzle over a little Nandos sauce

Add any extra vegetables that you like.

Tuna, Quinoa and Houmous with Watercress and Tomatoes *(Serves 1)*

Ingredients
½ sachet of precooked quinoa
1 tin of tuna
2 teaspoons of houmous
Handful of watercress (or chopped lettuce)
¼ onion – finely diced
5-6 cherry tomatoes sliced

Step 1
Open and drain the tuna.

Step 2
In a bowl stir the tuna through the quinoa.

Step 3
Put the watercress and sliced tomatoes on a plate and spoon the tuna/quinoa on the top.

Step 4
Add a blob of houmous on the top and sprinkle the chopped onion over the top.

Chicken Rice *(serves 1)*

Ingredients
¾ cup brown (basmati) rice
1 cup frozen peas
1 cup frozen sweetcorn
1 chicken breast
Olive oil
Nando's sauce

Step 1
Cook the rice as directed on the packet. Whilst the rice is cooking, dice the chicken breast and cook in a frying pan with a little olive oil.
Step 2
Once cooked, drain the rice in a colander and run under cold water to quickly cool the rice.
Step 3
In another saucepan put the peas and sweetcorn, cover with water and bring to the boil. Once boiling cook for a few minutes then drain off the water.
Step 4
Heat the rice in the microwave until piping hot, stir in the peas, sweetcorn and chicken, and drizzle some Nando's sauce over the top.

In a hurry!!
Use
1 sachet of brown rice
1 tin of peas
1 tin of sweetcorn
1 pre-cooked chicken breast or chicken leg
Heat the rice, peas, and sweetcorn in the microwave, mix together and drizzle some Nando's sauce over the top.
Serve with the chicken. If you choose to heat the chicken, make sure that it is cooked right through.

Egg Fried Rice (Serves 1)

Ingredients
1 sachet of wholegrain rice
2 eggs
1 cup of frozen peas
Tamari or soy sauce

Step 1
Cook the peas in a saucepan and drain the water off.
Whilst the peas are cooking put the rice in the microwave.

Step 2
Heat a small amount of olive oil in a frying pan.

Step 3
Crack the eggs into a cup and whisk a little with a fork, then add to the
frying pan. Stir the egg continuously until the egg forms a scrambled
egg consistency.

Step 4
Add the rice and peas to the frying pan and stir the egg through. Leave
to fry in the pan for a couple of minutes.
Add a sprinkle of tamari or soy sauce and stir through.

Bean Salad (serves 1-2)

Ingredients

1 tin of mixed beans
½ red onion - diced
2 tomatoes - diced
1/3 of a cucumber - diced
Small tin of sweetcorn
1 chilli - chopped

Step 1
Chop the onion, tomatoes, cucumber into small pieces.

Step 2
Open the beans and drain off the water, then wash them under the cold tap. Allow the water to drain off.

Step 3
In a bowl mix the onion, tomato, cucumber, and sweetcorn with the mixed beans.

Step 4
Add the chilli and serve.

Pitta Pizza *(serves 1-2)*

Ingredients
2 wholemeal pittas
Tomato puree or pesto
Vegetables of your choice diced into small pieces such as onions, peppers, and mushrooms.
Tinned sweetcorn (optional)
Jalapeno peppers
Tuna, cooked chicken, or ham
Grated cheese

Step 1
Pre heat the oven to 180°C
Place the pittas on a plate and spread a layer of tomato puree (or pesto) evenly on one side of the pitta.

Step 2
Sprinkle evenly a generous amount of diced vegetables on to the pitta.

Step 3
Add your choice of meat or fish or leave this step out if you are vegetarian.

Step 4
Add some sweetcorn and jalapeno peppers and finish with an even layer of grated cheese.

Step 5
Using a spatula, move the pizzas on to a baking tray and cook in the oven for approximately 15 minutes.

REALLY QUICK DINNERS

- Pasta with green or red pesto.
- Tinned curry with brown rice and a side salad.
- Omelette and salad.
- Soup with wholemeal bread.
- Scrambled egg on toast with watercress and tomatoes.
- Stir fry with nuts, chicken or edamame beans and brown rice noodles.
- Jacket potatoes and beans.
- Tinned soup (containing vegetables and rice, beans, or noodles to bulk it out) with 2 slices of wholemeal or seeded bread.
- Pre-prepared salad with smoked mackerel and wholemeal bread.

INDEX